Two weeks to a skinny you: Finally lose weight without dieting!

I0415295

by

Amelia Walkers

Copyright © 2012 Amelia Walkers

ISBN: 978-1-291-22264-7

www.publishnation.co.uk

Table of Contents

Introduction

- Vitamin A
- Vitamin D
- Vitamin E
- Vitamin K
- Vitamin C
- Vitamin B

7. All about minerals

- Calcium
- Iron
- Selenium
- Zinc
- Chromium
- Magnesium
- Manganese
- Copper

8. Fibre: An essential nutrient in your diet.

9. Weight loss v Fat loss: What is more important?

10. Vegetarian v Non-vegetarian: Which is better?

11. Do we need nutritional supplements?

12. Water and weight loss

13. Stimulants: Tea and coffee

14. Dieting: Your lifelong commitment

15. Effectiveness of some common diets:

- Weight loss pills
- Slimming tea
- Low carb diets
- High protein diets
- Low fat diets

16. The four simple rules to a new you!

17. Learn for life: Some simple guidelines!

Introduction

Losing weight, as you will realise by the end of the book (let's hope), is just the side-effect of following the simple rule of eating the right quantity of food at the right time. Miracle foods or crash diets are not a long term solution to weight loss. Through this book I share with you my weight loss journey and how I discovered the way to losing weight without dieting. Eating correctly has to be a lifelong commitment. Crash diets and miracle foods are not the answer to losing weight and staying healthy. What we eat should be planned according to our activity, lifestyle, fitness levels, likes and dislikes and so on.

We are all genetically prone to carry fat in different parts of our body (hence the apple or pear shaped bodies). However, the basics of fat loss and weight loss remain the same regardless of shape, size, gender, age or nationality. Most importantly, this book will teach you how to feel good about yourself and help you to understand that diet does not mean starvation. Once you understand that eating properly and exercising is the key to a happy and healthy life, you will automatically start losing weight and feel good about yourself.

About this book

This book will change your perception about dieting and urge you to think differently about your body and food. Once you read and follow the guidelines in the book, you will notice that you feel different in as little as one week. You will respect the food you eat, sleep better and have more energy. You will even drop a dress size in a month and will know automatically when your stomach is sending you the signal that it has now reached the overeating threshold. You will love your body and stop worrying about your weight.

My book is about my personal experience of losing weight in a simple and logical way. You will see that the first chapter talks about the three common complications associated with a poor lifestyle. I had an unhealthy lifestyle and was never exercising. I experienced all three of these complications at some point of my life and was able to get rid of all three by simply following the guidelines and rules in this book. You will see that by adopting the rules and guidelines in this book, I managed to not only lose so much weight in such a short time but I succeeded in conceiving (Now a healthy beautiful one year old baby girl) after being condemned by doctors. It all started …

Why did I want to lose the weight?

I have always hated my weight and have always been on some sort of diet for the last seven years in order to lose the weight. However, I was getting increasingly worried about my weight since both my parents were diagnosed with diabetes some five years ago. In 2010 after seven years of marriage my husband and I decided to try for a baby. We thought that now that my studies were over it was the right time. I was 26 and he was 29. Since I was having irregular periods (due to me putting on weight), we decided to consult a doctor to find out if we can do something about this. I did some tests and after one week

I was called by the doctor. I was simply told that I had PCOS and hence the weight gain. When asked what this meant about me conceiving, the doctor again simply said that I will have difficulty conceiving and even if successful there is a 75% chance I might miscarry. He told me that all this is due to my weight and unhealthy lifestyle which consisted of junk foods and no exercise. I felt so embarrassed about this and was in tears afterwards. Then I was pregnant thank God after a year due to modifying slightly my lifestyle. However, again in my pregnancy I started eating unhealthily under the pretext that I was eating for two. I was diagnosed with Gestational Diabetes in the eighth month of my pregnancy and was put on insulin for one week before being told that I had to undergo an induced birth. Finally, after the birth of my baby I was depressed with my look and again was relying on 'comfort eating' to the point that I started putting on more weight in a short time. I started having joint pains and hair loss. I was told to check for thyroid function by my doctor as he thought that this might be due to my thyroid not functioning properly. After that I knew I had to do something about my weight. I was sick and tired of being overweight. I felt like a 40-year old in a 26-year old body and was physically and mentally exhausted. I was sick and tired of struggling to do the basic things plus I just wanted to feel and look young again.

The three common complications associated with a poor lifestyle

Diabetes is a common life-long health condition. Diabetes is a condition where the amount of glucose in your blood is too high because the body cannot use it properly. This is because your pancreas does not produce any insulin, or not enough, to help glucose enter your body's cells – or the insulin that is produced does not work properly (known as insulin resistance). Insulin is the hormone produced by the pancreas that allows glucose to enter the body's cells, where it is used as fuel for energy so we can work, play and generally live our lives. It is vital for life.Glucose comes from digesting carbohydrate and is also produced by the liver. If you have diabetes, your body cannot make proper use of this glucose so it builds up in the blood and isn't able to be used as fuel. Your cells are starving. You should not skip carbohydrates for dinner but instead you should get the wholesome ones. The worst thing for diabetes is really low blood sugar. You should eat every two/three hours. Selenium, zinc and chromium will help your insulin respond better. Also, exercising will help stabilise blood sugar. A good and restful sleep will help the insulin function well.

Hypothyroid can affect anyone at any age, regardless of gender. With hypothyroid, your body's thyroid gland does not produce sufficient amounts of thyroid hormone, resulting in a slowed metabolic rate. The third largest endocrine gland in the body, the thyroid is a butterfly-shaped gland located below the voice box, wrapping around the trachea. It is responsible for producing the thyroid hormone essential to such bodily functions as growth, healthy energy levels and an optimal metabolic rate. A slow metabolism interferes with your body's ability to burn fat, so those with hypothyroidism often experience weight gain when their condition is not treated properly. Since your metabolism keeps muscles functioning properly, controls body temperature and is key in allowing you to properly digest and eliminate the food you eat, hypothyroidism can impair these essential metabolic processes. The weight gain can then lead to obesity, which carries its own serious health risks, including diabetes, heart disease and certain types of cancer. You should try to include some iodine-rich foods in your diet. Examples are bananas, carrots, strawberries, milk and whole grains. Also you should try to perform cardio exercises to improve mobility of fatty acids in your system. Remember that exercising regularly helps in reducing stress, improving the immune system function and metabolism. Sleeping well and waking up fresh are the key to the supporting the thyroid function.

Polycystic Ovary Syndrome (PCOS) occurs when the ovaries do not make enough hormones for the eggs to fully mature. Instead of releasing a mature egg during ovulation, some of the follicles in the ovaries turn into fluid-filled sacs called cysts. PCOS makes it more difficult for the body to use the hormone insulin, which normally helps convert sugars and starches from foods into energy. This condition, called insulin resistance, can cause insulin and sugar (glucose) to build up in the bloodstream. High insulin levels increase the production of male hormones called androgens. High androgen levels lead to symptoms such as body hair growth, acne, irregular periods and weight gain. Because the weight gain is triggered by male hormones, it is typically in the abdomen. That is where men tend to carry weight. So, instead of having a pear shape, women with PCOS have more of an apple shape. Abdominal fat is the most dangerous kind of fat. That's because it is associated with an increased risk of heart disease and other health conditions. You should lower your body fat levels to make easier for your ovaries to breathe. You should eat fresh and avoid over-heating food. You need unprocessed carbohydrates and proteins. You should go for the essential fatty acids like

Omega-3 and Omega-6 which help decrease the glycemic index of the food. Remember that you will need an abundant supply of vitamin B12 which is crucial for iron absorption (Low haemoglobin levels are always a factor with irregular periods and high body fat levels). Calcium is also required if you have PCOS. Do not forget that regular workouts are the key to regular periods.

Lifestyle Modification: Diet and exercise are important parts of managing the above conditions. Knowing the right foods to eat as well as the kinds of food to limit can improve the way you feel and help you lose weight, too. Eating well, staying active, and maintaining a healthy weight (or losing even a small amount of weight if you are overweight) can improve your health.

Weight loss v Fat loss: What is more important?

Weight loss and fat loss are not quite the same thing and you need to figure out which takes priority. People seem to use the terms weight loss and fat loss interchangeably, not understanding the difference between them. It is important, however, that you do understand -- there is a big difference between losing weight and losing fat. What's the difference? Let's start by defining weight loss and fat loss. Weight loss is the loss in your body weight -- the sum weight of your bones, muscles, organs, body fat and water in the body. Fat loss is the loss in your body fat -- the amount of fat your body carries. Healthy goals are 12-20 % body fat for men and 18-25 % for women. Weight is good, not bad; you do not want to lose weight, and more importantly for your health, you do not want to lose muscle. Our weight is made up of tissue, muscle, bone, blood, fat, water, and the rest of our physical bodies. Muscle, like every other component of our physical make-up, is most important. And fat is also a necessary, vital part of our physical make-up. Excess fat, however, is bad news and that is what you should focus on -- fat loss. Every time you talk about weight loss, what you are actually trying to achieve is fat loss. When you start eating healthy and exercising regularly, you will initially see a drop in your body fat but not as much in your weight.

All about carbs

Carbohydrates fall into two major categories: simple (including sugar, honey and maple syrup) and complex (including whole grains, starchy vegetables and legumes). Carbohydrates are responsible for providing our body with the energy it needs for normal day to day functioning. Most importantly, carbohydrates help in the functioning of our brain cells and neurons. The body is able to carry out its functioning without carbohydrates but it cannot think without carbs. If you care about your health eat your carbs. Just be careful to choose slow carbs. Carbs that retain their fibre are low on GI. The blood sugar (glucose) that is delivered to the cells throughout our bodies via our bloodstream is partly derived from the carbohydrates in the foods that we eat. A food with a low glycaemic index (GI) typically raises blood sugar levels only moderately, while a food with a high GI may cause blood sugar levels to increase more than desired. When we look at the GI figures associated with various carbohydrates, we find that some of the foods traditionally classified as complex carbohydrates - such as peeled, boiled potatoes - can increase our blood sugar levels more rapidly than some of the simple carbohydrates like table sugar! Because GI values can help us predict the functional effects in our bodies of the carbohydrates we eat, the GI has become an important tool for helping us select the right foods to help stabilize our blood sugar levels.

The Glycaemic Index

The Glycaemic Index (GI) is a numerical scale used to indicate how fast and how high a particular food can raise our blood glucose (blood sugar) level. A food with a low GI will typically prompt a moderate rise in blood glucose, while a food with a high GI may cause our blood glucose level to increase above the optimal level. Your body can take high GI food only after exercise, when your body needs instant sugar. Just because it's good for you don't eat all you want; always keep in touch with your stomach and make sure you do not cross the overeating threshold.Processed food leads to dullness and lethargy.Some diets so severely restricted carbs that it interfered with dieters' day to day functioning and thinking. So eat high fibre carbohydrates as much as possible and cut biscuits, cakes, pastries, pizzas and anything that's low fibre. Type 2 diabetes can be managed very easily by reducing the glycaemic load at one time; i.e. eating small portions many times a day and consuming slow or low GI carbs. Sweets and desserts are high on the glycaemic index because they are high in everything that is processed; sugar and flour.So eat your pizza, but stop at one piece. Where the glycaemic index is very high, reduce the load. The best time to eat high GI food is post exercise. We should eat fruit when we are in a fasting state or when our liver store is empty; so, first thing in the morning on an empty stomach, or immediately after physical exercise. So eat your fruit first thing in the morning – but before your breakfast, not with it. Alcohol is treated as foreign substance by the body.If you must drink, drink no more than once a week, and always after food (or with it but never on an empty stomach) and with at least a glass of water.Post exercise the body is in need of some fast carbs (the only time that the body needs high glycaemic index carbohydrate is post exercise) and a quick supply of amino acids.

All about proteins

The primary function of protein is to build and repair your body. Protein is important for maintaining muscle and bone mass, for keeping the immune system strong, and to prevent fatigue.Proteins are made out of chains of amino acids. Some amino acids can be made by the body (generally from other amino acids), but some cannot. The ones that cannot are known as "essential" or "indispensable."Twenty amino acids are used to build protein, but they are not the only amino acids.

High protein diets only replace your carbohydrate and fat sources with protein rich foods. There is no way of knowing whether you are reaching your daily requirement of protein. And in case you are reaching your daily requirement of protein, then in the absence of carbs and fat it will be rendered useless. For protein to work as it is supposed to, the body should get its supply of carbohydrate and fat. When too much of protein is consumed at one time, it does not get stacked away for future use; instead it is converted to fat by a process called deamination. Low protein diet is also not good. When we are deprived of a nutrient like protein, weight loss occurs only because the body breaks down its muscle to make up for the resultant lack of amino acids.

Consume an adequate protein diet and eat a diet with balanced amounts of carbohydrate and fat so that protein is free to perform its primary functions. Increasing activity without increasing protein only leads to muscle wasting. Protein is found in all meat, fish, egg, legumes, milk and milk products and soy.

Avoid red meat (too much of saturated fats) or at least restrict it to no more than once a week. Fish and eggs are better than chicken; fish is a rich source of omega -3 fatty acids. Most proteins need to be cooked well as it makes it easier on your stomach. This applies to all meats, egg and pulses. Only fish and dairy products can be eaten raw.

Vegetarian v Non-vegetarian: Which is better?

In the eternal debate of which is better vegetarian or non-vegetarian, we need to look at protein. The idea behind vegetarianism is that of non-violence or compassion towards all. Too much food is a form of cruelty too; you are cruel to your own stomach. There is enough evidence to show that the human digestive system is better suited for vegetarian food. However, vegetarian or non-vegetarian, the decision depends on various factors such as cultural or dietary habits of the family, personal preference, taste and avoidance of certain foods for health reasons. Our body's ability to digest and absorb proteins depends on our state of mind, time of the day and most importantly on how full we are feeling. Vegetarian or non-vegetarian, whatever you choose, be kind to yourself and your stomach and eat only a little at one time.

All about fats

Fat plays a big role in our body. Fats provide energy. Each gram of fat provides nine calories of energy for the body, compared with four calories per gram of carbohydrates and proteins.Fats build healthy cells - Fats are a vital part of the membrane that surrounds each cell of the body. Without a healthy cell membrane, the rest of the cell couldn't function.Fats build brains - Fat provides the structural components not only of cell membranes in the brain, but also of myelin, the fatty insulating sheath that surrounds each nerve fiber, enabling it to carry messages faster.Fats help the body use vitamins - Vitamins A, D, E, and K are fat-soluble vitamins, meaning that the fat in foods helps the intestines absorb these vitamins into the body.Fats make hormones - Fats are structural components of some of the most important substances in the body, including prostaglandins, hormone-like substances that regulate many of the body's functions. Fats regulate the production of sex hormones, which explains why some teenage girls who are too lean experience delayed pubertal development and amenorrhea.Fat provides healthier skin - One of the more obvious signs of fatty acid deficiency is dry, flaky skin. In addition to giving skin its rounded appeal, the layer of fat just beneath the skin (called subcutaneous fat) acts as the body's own insulation to help regulate body temperature. Lean people tend to be more sensitive to cold; obese people tend to be more sensitive to warm weather.Fat forms a protective cushion for your organs. Many of the vital organs, especially the kidneys, heart, and intestines are cushioned by fat that helps protect them from injury and hold them in place. So eat fat to lose fat.

Now there are many types of fat, each one having a specific role to play in the body.

These can be divided in the following categories:

Saturated fats: These are solid at room temperature: butter, animal fats (especially red meat), milk and milk products, coconut and palm oil. Long chain fatty acids are found in animal fats. These damage cardiovascular health and are hard to digest. Ghee (which is basically clarified butter obtained after milk is taken through a process of curdling and heating, or clarifying) has short chain fatty acids. These are easy to digest and promote good health.As a general rule, the fats in animal fats are tough on the body, while the ones found in dairy products are easily absorbed. Include healthy fats in your diet, like nuts (including peanuts), cheese, ghee, paneer and fish.

Unsaturated fats: These are fats which are liquid at room temperature; so all oils except for coconut oil. Fat has essential fatty acids. Unsaturated fats are further divided into three groups.

<u>Mono Unsaturated Fatty Acids (MUFA)</u> is found in peanuts, olives, avocados, almonds. They are considered very crucial in maintaining the health of the heart. The popularity of olive oil has grown tremendously in the last few years, as the people's sense of how healthy it is.

<u>Poly Unsaturated Fatty Acids (PUFA)</u> comes in two types: omega 3 and omega 6. Omega 6 is found in sunflower, safflower and soy bean oils. Omega 3 is found in flax seed, walnuts and the oils in fish. These fats have heart protecting values too.

<u>Trans fats</u>are created to preserve food and give it texture. They are made by converting unsaturated fats into saturated fats, by a process called hydrogenation. Trans fats are commonly used by restaurants, fast food chains and companies that produce food on a large scale and for commercial purposes, as it is cheaper. Most processed foods, store-bought cakes, biscuits and fast food such as pizzas, burgers, and fries have this kind of fat. This is the bad fat as it increases the levels of low

density lipo-protein or bad cholesterol in our body. We should avoid this fat.

All about vitamins

Vitamins and minerals make your body work properly. Vitamins fall into two categories: fat soluble and water soluble. The fat-soluble vitamins - A, D, E, and K - dissolve in fat and can be stored in your body. The water-soluble vitamins - C and the B-complex vitamins [such as vitamins B6 (pyridoxine), B12 (cobalamin), B3 (niacin), B2 (riboflavin), B1 (thiamin) B5 (pantothenic acid), B7 (biotin) and B9 (folic acid) — need to dissolve in water before your body can absorb them. They do not provide our body with any energy or calories but they are important so that we can use our energy or calories well.

Vitamin A is found in whole and low fat milk, dark leafy vegetables, all the orange, yellow vegetables and in the liver and kidney. We need it because it supports our immune functions, helps improve eyesight, is crucial for the growth and development of our body, and is a potent antioxidant which protects cells against free radical. Vitamin A should be taken when you are stressed or travelling.

<u>Vitamin D</u> is found in our body upon exposure to sunlight. We can also get this vitamin from fish and egg yolks. It aids calcium absorption. A deficiency in vitamin D would manifest itself in bowing of legs, curving of spine, loss of bone density, joint pain and discomfort.

<u>Vitamin E</u> is found in polyunsaturated vegetable oils like corn, soy, sunflower, safflower oil and seeds, nuts, whole grains. Asparagus, green leafy vegetables, berries and tomatoes are good sources of this one. We need it because it protects the heart, keeps the skin young, prevents nerve and muscular weakness and is a powerful oxidant. We should take it when we have eaten a lot of fried food, bakery products and consumed high amounts of fat.

<u>Vitamin K</u> is found in green leafy vegetables, green peas, green tea, oats, and whole grain.

This vitamin plays a major role in blood clotting and is important in preventing and treating osteoporosis, and for building healthy bones. One should take it if suffering from excessive menstrual blood.

Vitamin C is found in most fruits and vegetables. We need it because it is critical to our immunity, helps manufacture hormones, collagen, maintains our respiratory system and lung function and is a powerful antioxidant. Vitamin C also protects us against heart disease, has a supporting function of vitamin E in the body, and protects sperms from damage.

Vitamin B is found in fresh fruits, vegetables, whole grains, nuts, eggs, fish and cheese. We need it because it takes part in metabolic reactions, helps metabolise carbohydrates, aids digestion, improves nerve function and prevents depression. We should take it as a supplement at the start of the day with our breakfast so that we can utilize nutrients better throughout the day.

Fibre: An essential nutrient in your diet.

Fibre is an important part of a healthy balanced diet and it contains no calories or vitamins. The main function of fibre is to keep the digestive system healthy and functioning properly by helping the digestive system to process food and absorb nutrients. Fibre aids and speeds up the excretion of waste and toxins from the body. Fibre can help to lower blood cholesterol and makeus feel fuller and so help to control our appetite.There are two types of fibre: insoluble and soluble. Insoluble fibre helps the bowel to pass food by making stools soft and bulky thus preventing constipation.Insoluble fibre is found in foods like beans, brown rice, fruits with edible seeds, maize, oats, pulses, wholegrain. Soluble fibre lowers cholesterol levels and controls blood sugar. It can be found in all fruit and vegetables.

All about minerals

Calcium is found in dairy products, tofu, green leafy vegetables, nuts, seeds and in almost all wholesome food. We need it because it maintains the health of bones, joints, and teeth, is responsible for all muscular contraction, for clotting of blood and to regulate blood pressure. We should take it as a supplement every day.

Iron is found in meat, fish, egg, whole grains, fresh vegetables and fruits. Iron is a part of haemoglobin which transports oxygen from lungs to different tissues of the body and carbon dioxide from different tissues to the lungs.

Selenium, zinc, chromium, magnesium, manganese and copper are found in fish, egg, whole grains and fresh vegetables. These minerals are essential in preventing diseases and they are antioxidants. They promote fat burning in the body and help improve insulin sensitivity. Zinc and chromium are important for good skin and hair growth and to prevent acne and wrinkles. Zinc also helps in normal testosterone function and aids muscle growth. Selenium protects us against free radicals. Copper, on the other hand, is needed for optimum iron absorption whilst manganese is responsible for thyroid function and blood sugar control. Magnesium helps lower blood pressure, eases PMS symptoms and lowers LDL levels.

Dieting: Your lifelong commitment.

The word diet has been wrongly interpreted by many people. We hear that manypeople go on crash or extreme diets in order to lose weight. If you look at the definition of crash diet in Wikipedia, it says: 'A crash diet is a diet which is extreme in its nutritional deprivations, typically severely restricting calorie intake. It is meant to achieve rapid weight loss and may differ from outright starvation only slightly. They are not meant to last for long periods of time, at most a few weeks. Importantly, the term specifically implies a lack of concern for proper nutrition. Extreme diets are not sustainable and just do not work. The minute we are 'off' the diet all our weight is back.

However, dieting is not about starving but about eating well, eating right and eating regularly. We should eat the right amount of food at the right time. We should not go on a diet just to lose weight because we have this special occasion coming or we want this smaller dress size to fit us. Eating correctly has to be a lifelong commitment.What is most important is that you feel good about yourself, commit to eating properly and exercising; and weight loss, rather fat loss, will just happen.Dieting or eating correctly is a process. Diet is not starvation. It has to be a representation of what you will be eating your entire life. You can overeat sometimes; this is not the end of the world. Just get back to your good eating habit now. Instead of going on a diet we need to modify our lifestyle and eat the right quantity at the right time.

Stimulants: Tea and coffee

People drink coffeeand teaall over the world. In some countries coffee is drunk up to five times a day. But sometimes these stimulants can cause serious damage to health. You should not have tea or coffee first thing in the morning on an empty stomach. You have to make sure that you eat something before that. When we sleep, our blood sugar levels drop in the night. In the morning our liver stores are almost empty. So our blood sugar is low. Low blood sugar is also a reason why we feel 'low' in the morning. The body sometime takes to wasting or breaking our muscle down to keep our sugar from dropping to abnormally low levels. Similarly, if you are tired and have not eaten for some time or have just overeaten, your blood sugar first suddenly increases, and then dramatically decreases; you feel depressed, lethargic and need something to cheer up. This effect is given by hormoneadrenalin, which is emitted by the adrenal gland.

Stimulants like tea or coffee, which has caffeine, jolt the system out of slumber. It increases the blood pressure, heart rate, breathing rate and makes the body feel stressed or 'kicked' like we say. We mistake this for feeling awake. In reality, the body experiences stress because of the increase in its heart and breathing rate and will respond by hampering fat burning. Stress is the biggest enemy of an efficient digestive system and of the fat burning processes of the body. If the organism is stressed for a long period of time, the adrenal gland starts to emit cortisol, which destroys the nervous system. Also, stimulants upset the balance of the blood glucose and thus enhance the resistance to insulin with controls the blood sugar level. As a result, this provokes excess weight and fatigue. For instance, many people like to have a cup of coffee after dinner. However, what they do not know is that the coffee will come in the way of their sleep and it will interfere with the digestion and make the stomach acidic so they wake up bloated and constipated. With a disturbed metabolism, the body starts to store fat.

What is the solution? Simple. To be able to burn fat effectively, we have to train our body to preserve lean tissue, i.e. muscle; not waste it by breaking it down into glucose to keep your blood sugar up. To do this we must eat real food instead of consuming these stimulants to curb our hunger. We have to eat something that will lead to a slow, steady increase in our blood sugar levels. This balances the insulin in the body and helps our hungry cells to get the nutrients that it is craving for. Similarly, when we wake up in the morning the heart and breathing rates are at its lowest as this reflects a relaxed state of mind and body. To keep the system relaxed, we need to give it real food, which is easy on the heart, lungs and stomach too. Both if we have coffee or tea first thing when we wake up then there will be an increase in our blood sugar levels and the cells will still be starved since they have been without nutrition for the last 8 to 10 hours since we had dinner the night before.

Water and weight loss

Water is the most important nutrient in your body. It is the primary transporter in the body. About 70% of the human body is water. Our lifestyle is dehydrating since we consume too much of processed food, drink too much caffeine, sugary drinks and wine. Even a small drop in the water content of the body lowers our blood volume which in turn causes a reduction in the supply of oxygen to our muscles as a result we will feel tired. This increases the sodium content in our blood which triggers the thirst response. Most of us drink water only to quench our thirst rather than to meet our body's water requirement. As a result we are dehydrated. A dehydrated body means our kidneys find it difficult processing our wastes which can in turn poison our system. Muscles cannot contract, the joints will hurt, the skin will look dull, the lungs cannot breath and the heart cannot beat without water. Also, fat loss will be impaired without adequate water.

We should be drinking enough water (try 6 to 8 glasses daily) so that our urine is always crystal clear, not light yellow, dark yellow or reddish. Since we lose water in many ways like through urine, excretion, sweat, breathing; we can hydrate ourselves by sipping water throughout the day and eat wholesome unprocessed food. Remember that water is life and a blessing!

Extreme or crash diets affect the water reserves in our body. These diets lead to a rapid water loss (instead of weight loss) from the body. The drop in the body weight as a result of such diets is due to water loss and not fat loss. Loss of water in the body will impair circulation, reduce muscle tone, joint, bone and thus overload the kidney, lungs and heart. And this will also lead to body odour since the composition of sweat changes. Would you prefer losing the all-important water in your body just to be happy with the scale?

A study from the University of North Carolina at Chapel Hill Research shows that, in fact, people who drink an average of 6½ cups (52 ounces) of water each day consume 200 fewer calories a day. Let's analyse this a little more. 200 less calories is about 73,000 fewer calories in a year and it takes 3,500 calories to create 1 pound of fat. This means you're losing about 20 extra pounds of fat a year.The process of burning calories requires an adequate supply of water in order to function efficiently as dehydration slows down the fat-burning process. The burning calories create toxins and water plays animportant role in flushing them out of the body. No doubt drinking water with a meal will make you feel full sooner and therefore satisfied eating less.

Do we need nutritional supplements?

This short answer to this question is "Yes!" In an ideal world, we would not need health supplements. We have hectic lifestyles and thus find it difficult to consume the nutrients our body need every day. Even if you make sure that you are eating healthily, there may be factors beyond our control. So, why do we think that a healthy diet may still not provide us with adequate vitamins and minerals?

Our soil is contaminated and lacks minerals such as zinc and selenium. This is because of poor farming methods, the use of synthetic fertilisers and ecological factors. The depletion in these two minerals has increased the risk of heart disease and cancer. Statistics show that death from lung cancer, cervix, breast, rectum, bladder and oesophagus cancer rise concurrently in counties with lower levels of selenium. In a report published in "The Journal of the American College of Nutrition", evidence shows reduced levels of six valuable nutrients examined in vegetables and fruits, grown in mineral-deficient soils. These include: vitamin C, potassium, iron, calcium, protein and riboflavin. Researchers at University of Texas reported a steady decline in vitamins and minerals in US soil from the 1950s to present.

Our fruits are covered with pesticides and injected with glucose, polished with wax. The methods commercial fruits and vegetables are ripened are questionable. For instance, in order to prevent bruising, some fruits are shipped while they are still green. They are then left to ripen for days to weeks. Ethylene gas which would normally be produced naturally by a fruit at the correct time will be artificially applied instead. As a result the fruits become carcinogenic and contain arsenic. Moreover, some people use insecticides or kerosene to hasten the ripening process. Artificial ripening processes can lead to neurological disorders.

Studies have also shown that premature picking of vegetables and fruits results in loss of important nutrients. For instance, a comprehensive study of cherries by Spain researchers showed a 50% loss of vitamin C when they are picked prematurely. Similarly, a studyconducted by the Oregon State University researchers concluded that when blackberries are picked while green, they contained 243mg anthocyanin (antioxidant flavonoids) less than when they are ripened on the vine. Also, polyphenols (antioxidants from plant foods) do not develop properly when plants are prematurely picked and carotenoids (precursor to vitamin A antioxidants) are washed-out when tomatoes are prematurely picked, as they receive inadequate sunlight.

The way we cook and store our foods also contribute to the loss of important nutrients. When fresh or canned foods are processed, frozen or cooked, healthy vitamins are destroyed. For instance, during the sterilization process, canned meats and vegetables are subject to lose 50-100% of their vitamin A content. Even more shocking, all vitamin A is lost after 3-5 years in storage, according to one study.And the way we store grains, fruits and vegetables in big malls is disgusting.

Supplement is a necessity I would say. Vitamin and mineral supplements are no replacement to healthy eating, regular exercise and a positive attitude with restful sleep. However, they can help to balance an unhealthy diet. The stress that we experience is a major reason for nutrient depletion in our diet. We need supplements for vitamins like A, E, B and C and minerals like selenium, zinc, chromium and calcium.

Effectiveness of some common diets

Weight loss pills

Weight loss or diet pills are for some of us the answer to a quick loss of weight. However, the risks of these pills outweigh their benefits as a weight loss aid. While some side effects may seem minor and worth the risk, some side effects are very dangerous and can even be deadly. Natural herbal diet pills carry much the same risk as prescription or other diet pills do. In fact, some can even be more dangerous. For instance, you have probably heard of ephedra (ma huang). Ephedra was actually banned from the market because of the horrible side effects that users experienced and the cases of death. Yet, you can still get ephedra in tea products and on the internet. Some prescription drugs, although safer because they are FDA approved, can and often do, have very dangerous side effects. It is always advised to check with your doctor about the harmful consequences of taking a weight loss pill. The greatest danger of taking diet pills is that many of them may cause emotional and physical dependence. Moreover, weight loss pills can also seriously disrupt your natural metabolism. Most prescription diet pills suppress the appetite, which causes you to consume fewer calories. At first, this seems like the ultimate solution to losing unwanted pounds. However, as you reduce your caloric intake, your metabolism also slows down. As your metabolism slows, the amount of weight you lose also slows to a crawl. Suddenly it is harder to lose weight than ever, whether you are taking the drug or not! This is why it is common for people to lose only a certain amount of weight while taking diet pills alone. Furthermore, several over-the-counter diet pills have also been associated with health risks. For example, weight loss pills containing Ephedra increase the possibility of stroke, raised heart rate, high blood pressure, seizures or heart attack.

Slimming tea

Slimming tea has become the latest diet fad sweeping the nation. Whilst there are some scientifically proven benefits to drinking pure teas, there are many health risks that come from abuse or from occasional use of slimming teas. Weight loss teas come in a wide variety of brands. There are some studies that show that some slimming teas work by boosting the metabolism, suppressing the appetite, and by helping your body burn more calories through thermogenesis. These results are small and can happen with green tea for example. However, most slimming teas contain herbal laxatives which can cause you to go to the bathroom more often or even cause diarrhoea. Your body will drop water weight temporarily because your body flushes the water out of your system but you will also dump important nutrients from your body or get dehydrated. Many of the herbal teas advertised as fat burning or those that claim remarkable weight loss often contain sienna, a product that is mainly used as a laxative. The use of sienna for weight loss can be highly dangerous. In fact, this particular herb is often a prescribed laxative for those people who are severely constipated and have found no relief from stool softeners. Abuse of laxatives for fat burning or weight loss can cause the person to become dehydrated and can create problems in the gastric-intestinal tract. In fact, abuse can cause death.

Low carb diet

A low-carb diet limits carbohydrates. Many types of low-carb diets exist, each with varying restrictions on the types and amounts of carbohydrates you can eat. Atkins and South Beach diets are two examples of low-carb diets which are very famous worldwide. The theory behind the low-carb diet is that insulin prevents fat breakdown in the body by allowing sugar to be used for energy. Followers of the low-carb diet believe that decreasing carbs results in lower insulin levels, which causes the body to burn stored fat for energy and ultimately helps them shed excess weight and reduce risk factors for a variety of health conditions.

However, these diets so severely restrict carbs that it interfered with dieters' day to day functioning and thinking. Low carb diets lead to depletion of serotonin which is a neurotransmitter in the brain responsible for feeling of wellbeing, happiness and satisfaction. Low carb diets have been known to make dieters' moods off. Furthermore, if you suddenly and drastically cut carbs, you may experience a variety of temporary health effects, including headache, dizziness, weakness, fatigue and constipation.

In addition, some diets restrict carbohydrate intake so much that they can result in nutritional deficiencies. This can cause such health problems as constipation, diarrhoea and nausea. It is also possible that severely restricting carbohydrates to less than 20 grams a day can result in ketosis. Ketosis occurs when you do not have enough sugar (glucose) for energy, so your body breaks down stored fat, causing ketones to build up in your body. Side effects from ketosis can include nausea, headache, mental fatigue and bad breath.

Irritability restlessness, depression and anxiety are also common with some low-carb diets. Most low-carb diets promote high protein or fat in food. Some health experts believe that if you eat large amounts of fat and protein from animal sources your risk of heart disease or certain cancers may increase.

High protein diet

High protein diets promote high protein content in foods and can help you feel full longer and stabilize your blood sugar levels, but they also carry certain risks. Research shows that people who eat high protein diets based on meat have a higher rate of bone density loss. In the long run, bone density loss leads to osteoporosis. Doctors believe that the reason for this is that a high protein diet requires your body to process more calcium. While many high protein diets allow for the consumption of dairy products like milk, cheese and yogurt, your body might still extract calcium from your bones to get the extra amounts it needs to process the high amounts of protein in your diet.

It is also known that high protein diets can put strain on your kidneys. Your kidneys are responsible for filtering a number of substances, including protein, from your blood. So a high protein diet can put strain on your kidneys. Also, some studies show that high protein diets may contribute to the development of some cancers. Finally, one of the most common risks of high protein diets is nutritional deficiency.

Low fat diet

Eating a low fat diet has long been associated with good health, weight losing, reducing risk of developing life-threatening heart diseases and multiple health issues. However, fat is not entirely evil; a certain amount of fat is critical to our bodily functions. It regulates body temperature, cushions and insulates organs and tissues. As the most concentrated source of calories (nine calories per gram of fat compared with four calories per gram for protein and carbohydrates), fat is the main form of our body's energy storage.

Eating a diet too low in fat can interfere with the absorption of the fat-soluble vitamins A,

D, E and K. Because these nutrients are fat soluble, your body needs dietary fat to use them. These vitamins are stored mostly in the liver and fat tissue and are important in bodily functions such as growth, immunity, cell repair and blood clotting. If we restrict fat in our body, these vitamins will be excreted and you may be at risk of a vitamin deficiency.

Furthermore, a diet that is too low in fat (particularly omega-3s) can cause colon, breast, and prostate cancer. Research has shown that a high intake of omega-3s slows prostate tumour and cancer cell growth. Low-fat diets also play a role in cholesterol levels and heart disease. When your diet is too low in fat, your body's level of HDL (the "good" cholesterol) goes down. This is problematic because you want your HDL level to be high to help protect against heart disease. HDL collects "bad" cholesterol from the blood and transports it to the liver for excretion. When those ratios are out of balance—and when your LDL ("bad" cholesterol) level gets too high, you face cholesterol problems and an increased risk of heart disease. Essential fatty acids, especially Omega-3s, can elevate HDL, improve cholesterol levels and protect the heart.

Finally, if you are always choosing low-fat or fat-free foods at the grocery store, you could be hindering your weight-loss efforts. A lot of the so called 'low fat' is a waste of money. Why spend ridiculously high amounts to buy low fat foods when they contain only about 1 or max 2 grams of fat less than the regular 'full fat' varieties. Research has shown that people tend to believe these foods are "freebies' and will even overeat them, thinking they are healthy or low in calories. For instance, low fat ice creams are loaded with sugar or sweeteners and low fat chips are usually high in salt and are often baked and contain trans-fat which is responsible for the hardening of arteries, increasing body fat and causing many other health problems.

The four simple rules to a new you!

Rule 1

Eat real food within 30 minutes of waking up or as soon as possible.

Now that you know the harm that tea or coffee causes to your health when you have them first thing in the morning, you shouldaim to eat real food as soon as you wake up or within 30 minutes of waking up. Going hungry in the morning is a disaster for anybody who dreams of a healthy lifestyle and slim body. By not eating in the morning a huge calorie deficit is created in the morning and then the body has no other option but to overeat later to make up for that deficit. So when we feel like not having anything in the morning then we are definitely having a slow metabolic rate and a digestive system which is not functioning effectively. Breakfast is the most important meal of the day I would say, as it breaks the night long fast our body has been through. It also helps to improve the body's metabolism. Unfortunately, it is the one meal that people are most likely to miss each day because they are in a rush whilst others miss breakfast in an effort to lose weight. The metabolism is slower in people who miss breakfast, which can actually hinder a person from losing weight, rather than help them.

Many studies have shown how a full healthy breakfast can increase our metabolic rate.With sunrise, the metabolism peaks and the cells demand nutrition. This is the time to eat and to eat big. If you are not used to eating anything in the morning, no problem you can just have a fruit and later have your normal food like porridge, oatmeal, most egg dishes (scrambled, boiled, poached, omelettes). hot and cold cereals, roti, bread, shakes, homemade sandwich or anything that is healthy and rich in fibre. Note that those who feel like going to the loo first thing in the morning even before they eat or drink anything are on the right tract to healthy eating.

Eating early improves metabolic rate and reduces hunger pangs in the day. This is the best time to have a multivitamin as well. Eating first thing in the morning will lead to an increase in blood sugar and energy levels. This will lead to an increase in metabolic rate and fat burning and a decrease in acidity and bloating. By having a hearty breakfast in the morning you will not feel like overeating later in the day and you will have a stabilised blood sugar levels throughout the day which means you will have less chances of getting fat.

Advice: You should wake up closer to or before sunrise. Not only will you experience the peace that every dawn brings and pray leisurely and feel good about yourself, sunrise also provides us with vitamin D to maintain healthy bones.

Rule 2

Eat every 2 to 3 hours after your first meal.

By eating this way, you will effortlessly speed up your metabolism. Eating every two to three hours keeps your body from storing many calories as fat because it has a constant supply of food to use as energy. Your metabolism remains elevated and your blood sugar stable. Eating every 2 to 3 hours feeds muscle and starves fat. By eating frequently, you reassure your body that you aren't going to starve; that food will always be available. In addition, if your meals are spaced five or six hours apart, you may be prone to swings in hunger, which might cause overeating during or between meals.

Our stomach keeps secreting hydrochloric acid and keeps asking you to eat. But what we usually do is to either give it a tea, coffee, cigarette, mint or chewing gum, etc. and almost always choose not to eat, trying to starve off those hunger pangs as long as possible. When the hunger signal becomes unbearable we finally suffocate the stomach with so much food that we progressively work at weakening it; and therefore the hunger signals that it can send to our brain. Eating frequent meals every 2 to 3 hours is not just better for our digestive system, but it keeps us from overeating.

But when you adopt the idea of eating frequently, often what drops first is the size of the meal. When you eat every 3 hours a day, it's a given that you will eat small. When our body gets a regular dose of a small number of calories often, through the day, it feels reassured and loved. Eating is a way of loving our body and providing it with nourishment. When our body gets fewer calories at a time, they are utilised better and not stored as fat. Also, because the body is feeling reassured with a regular intake of calories and nutrients, it sees no reason to store body fat. The body loses fear of death due to starvation (which is instilled by a combination of long gaps between meals and eating a lot at one time), and feels encouraged to let go of its fat stores (which it has been holding on to as its means of survival).

Example

A daily plan might include a fruit for your first meal, any healthy meal for your breakfast within 1 hour of having your fruit. After that you can have a bowl of yogurt for your third meal, then your lunch as a fourth meal (rice + curry + salad or any other combination you like), a handful of roasted peanuts or 8-10 raw almonds as your fifth meal, dinner as your sixth meal and a glass of Jasmine Tea as your final meal.

Some people might have six meals a day whilst some others might be having eight to nine meals day depending on the level of activity they do every day. What is important is that you should adjust the number of meals you are having per day based on the level of activity you a particular day. You should eat more when you are more active and less when you are less active. Low activity means any time you are passive, or quite inactive or not using your mental energies; watching a movie or TV, surfing the net, making small talk on the phone, checking emails, doing low intensive work, being driven around, going out to a party, napping, delegating work; in short any routine work. We need to increase the number of meals during high demand periods and cut down when relaxing.

Advice: Frequent eating does not mean snacking. All we are doing is taking our 3 main meals (breakfast, lunch and dinner), cutting the portions, and then adding some in between meals to these main meals.

Rule 3

Eat your last meal 2-3 hours before bedtime.

Digesting food is a calorie burner and work for the body. In the night, cells are naturally not very sensitive to energy or nutrients as they do not really need much so if you overload your stomach most of it will get wasted or converted to fat. Eating too close to bedtime raises your body temperature, increases blood sugar and insulin, prevents the release of melatonin, and cuts down on growth hormone release. All these factors interfere with the quality of your sleep and the natural fat-burning benefits of a good night's rest. Furthermore, sleep deprivation leads to more cravings and a greater likelihood of overeating the next day.

The worst thing we can do is to eat a lot and then sleep immediately. A good quality and peaceful sleep is important for losing fat. When we sleep, our body repairs cells, balances the hormones, rejuvenates the cells of our body, repairs the damage that we have put our cells through during the day and gets ready for the next day. Without a restful sleep, our hormones or lean tissue will not be able to support fat burning. Stress or disturbed sleep throw the hormones off balance, and depletes us of lean tissue (muscle breakdown and bones thinning), both of which hinder fat burning.

In the night, when we sleep, our system should feel free to do what it is supposed to do: repair wear and tear and rejuvenate. When we eat too late or immediately before bedtime, the food remains undigested in the intestines. The undigested food remains in the tract and bacteria act upon it. This can turn the healthiest of meals into toxins. These toxins lead to acidity, bloating, constipation, gain in body fat levels and appearance of stretch marks. When food is not getting digested properly, it can leave a bad smell in your mouth.

Advice: You should avoid the computer screen or TV before bed as the light stimulates your brain, making it harder to fall asleep. Dessert post dinner is bad and caffeine can stay in your body for a long time and make your stomach acidic so that you wake up bloated and constipated. The ideal time to sleep is between 10 to 10.30 pm.

Rule 4

Commit to some kind of exercise 30 to 45 minutes for 3 days a week at least: Exercise is a MUST!

Exercise and dieting are complementary to each other. Dieting without exercising may provide you with initial results. However, in the long-run your metabolism will slow down, causing your body to burn fewer calories, and eventually result in much more weight gain than where you initially started.

Any programme which discourages you from exercising is useless. Being on a diet might help us lose weight, but without exercise we lose our muscles and bone density. The least we can do is to exercise 30 to 45 minutes for 3 days a week. Exercise is a part of adopting a better lifestyle but it is NOT an alternative to eating right. The only way to lose body fat is to eat right and at the right time and to exercise regularly. Unless you exercise, you will never see enough of a result, despite all your good eating habits.

Exercise is a way to improve fitness, blood circulation, and to love the body. Which exercise we choose as means to keeping fit is a completely personal choice as all forms of exercise lead us to health, vitality and peace. No doubt the benefits of exercise go way beyond losing weight or losing inches. It improves muscle and bone density, heart and lung function, lower blood pressure, stabilise blood sugar and make us active, faster and stronger. Walking is good but only if it provides a challenge to your body. If you cannot talk at all while walking, this means that you are walking or running too fast. If you can sing, then you are too slow. If you are walking properly, you will only be able to talk with difficulty. The best is to try running for 30 minutes at a stretch or try running a couple of rounds instead of just walking. Or better we should do interval training: run for a while then walk and keep repeating this cycle. It is important to always invest in good shoes and stretch before and after the run.

Advice: Always have a post- workout meal of high GI and protein within 20 minutes of any exercise.

Learn for life: Some simple guidelines!

> ➤ Eat in silence and while enjoying your own company. Switch off the TV or mobile.
> ➤ Sip a glass of water while eating.

- ➢ Eat fresh food – Do not deep freeze cooked food.
- ➢ There are no such things as miracle foods.
- ➢ We should aim for fat loss rather than weight loss.
- ➢ Diet is not starvation.
- ➢ Everything that is herbal is not necessarily safe. You should consult a qualified herbalist or ayurvedic doctor to make sure that the herbal product matches your body constitution.
- ➢ Everything made in laboratories is not always dangerous and artificial.
- ➢ Exercise and dieting are not mutually exclusive.
- ➢ Any programme which says that you do not have to exercise to lose weight is worthless.
- ➢ Do not judge your health by the body mass index (BMI) because it is just about total body weight and do not consider the contribution of fat weight towards the total weight.

- Most low fat foods are barely 1 or 2 grams lower in fat than full fat versions but are sold at a more expensive price.
- Regular use of sweeteners is associated with certain type of cancers, acidity, obesity, thyroid malfunction, etc.
- Eat fruit as a meal in itself and not as a dessert after dinner.
- When it comes to fruit, eat rather than drink.
- According to Ayurveda, overeating (eating a large quality of food at the wrong time) is the cause of all diseases.
- Try not to store sweets or fried foods at home.
- Eat whole vegetables and fruits instead of cutting them as they lose vitamins from their surface.
- Never buy the pre-packed cut vegetables and fruits in the supermarkets.
- Wake up before or close to sunrise.
- Every calorie we consume should be loaded with nutrients.
- A relaxed state of mind is the best preparation for any indulgence.

- Make sure that the food you eat is not 'empty' and processed; that it is natural and full of goodness like cheese, peanuts, nuts, milk, yoghurt and whole grains.
- The key to eating right is to focus while you eat: switch off the TV and mobile phone.
- You can digest the most amount of food between 7 am and 10 am.
- Stress can make you fat.
- How many nutrients a food has is much more important than how many calories.
- Drink enough water so that your urine is always crystal clear, not light yellow, dark yellow or reddish.
- The only way to hydrate ourselves is by sipping water all the time and by eating wholesome unprocessed food.
- Limit deep-fried food but do not avoid it completely. Just make sure that you eat immediately upon frying.
- Eat your fruit first thing in the morning on an empty stomach.

- ➢ MODERATION is the key word: Eat the right quantity of food at the right time. Note that the stomach is actually the size of 2 palms and the food it can take at a time is the amount that fits in your 2 palms.

THE END

About the Author

Amelia Walkers is a Barrister-at-law and part-time life coach in the United Kingdom. She has completed her degree in law, her Masters' degree in International Business and Commercial Law and her Bar Professional Training Course in the United Kingdom. She has worked as a law lecturer in London and also completed a diploma in life. She decided to write about her weight loss journey to help others to better understand the long term approach to a healthy lifestyle. The 28-year-old thinks that if we all use our common sense and love our body by eating healthily and exercising regularly then we will never need to rely on the so-called fad diets or miracle foods.

www.ingramcontent.com/pod-product-compliance
Lightning Source LLC
Chambersburg PA
CBHW062116280526
45788CB00003B/1480